Name: Aba, Abina
Meaning: Born on Thursday
Gender: Girl

Name: Abal
Meaning: Wild Rose
Gender: Girl

Name: Abam
Meaning: Sister of Twins
Gender: Girl

Name: Aban
Meaning: Unknown
Gender: Boy

Name: Abdul
Meaning: Servant
Gender: Girl

Name: Abeeku, Abla
Meaning: Born on Wednesday
Gender: Boy

Name: Abena, Abina
Meaning: Born on Tuesday
Gender: Girl

Name: Abla
Meaning: Born on Wednesday
Gender: Girl

Name: Addae
Meaning: Morning Sun
Gender: Boy

Name: Adeben
Meaning: Twelfth Born
Gender: Boy

Name: Adika
Meaning: First Child from a Second Husband
Gender: Boy

Name: Adio
Meaning: Righteous
Gender: Boy

Name: Adjo, Adjua, Adwoa, Adzo
Meaning: Born on Monday
Gender: Girl

Name: Adofo
Meaning: Warrior
Gender: Boy

Name: Adom
Meaning: Help from God
Gender: Boy

Name: Aduke
Meaning: Cherished One
Gender: Boy

Name: Adusa
Meaning: Unknown
Gender: Boy

Name: Adwin
Meaning: Creative
Gender: Boy

Name: Afafa
Meaning: First Child from a Second Husband
Gender: Girl

Name: Afi, Afua
Meaning: Born on Friday
Gender: Girl

Name: Afram
Meaning: Of the River
Gender: Boy

Name: Africa
Meaning: Sunny
Gender: Girl

Name: Afryea
Meaning: Born during Happy Times
Gender: Girl

Name: Afton
Meaning: Unknown
Gender: Girl

Name: Agape
Meaning: Lover
Gender: Girl

Name: Agwe
Meaning: Of the Sea
Gender: Girl

Name: Agyei
Meaning: Message from God
Gender: Boy

Name: Agyemang
Meaning: Unknown
Gender: Boy

Name: Agymah
Meaning: He Shall Leave Us
Gender: Boy

Name: Aiida
Meaning: Serene
Gender: Girl

Name: A'ishah
Meaning: Prosperous
Gender: Girl

Name: Akoni
Meaning: Courageous
Gender: Boy

Name: Akosua
Meaning: Born on Sunday
Gender: Girl

Name: Akwasi
Meaning: Born on Sunday
Gender: Boy

Name: Akwete
Meaning: Older Twin
Gender: Girl

Name: Akwetee
Meaning: Younger Twin
Gender: Boy

Name: Akwokwo
Meaning: Younger Twin
Gender: Girl

Name: Alizabeth
Meaning: Gift from God
Gender: Boy

Name: Alonsa
Meaning: Noble
Gender: Girl

Name: Alvina
Meaning: Friend of the Elves
Gender: Girl

Name: Alvita
Meaning: Vivacious
Gender: Girl

Name: Alyshia
Meaning: Honest
Gender: Girl

Name: Alvita
Meaning: Vivacious
Gender: Girl

Name: Ama
Meaning: Born on Saturday
Gender: Girl

Name: Amancia
Meaning: Lover
Gender: Girl

Name: Ametefe
Meaning: Born after his Father's Death
Gender: Boy

Name: Amin, Ameen
Meaning: Faithful
Gender: Boy

Name: Amir, Ameer
Meaning: Prince
Gender: Boy

Name: Amoa
Meaning: Unknown
Gender: Boy

Name: Amoani
Meaning: Unknown
Gender: Boy

Name: Amoy
Meaning: Goddess
Gender: Girl

Name: Ampah
Meaning: Trust
Gender: Boy

Name: Anan, Anane
Meaning: Fourth Son
Gender: Boy

Name: Anbarin
Meaning: Unknown
Gender: Girl

Name: Anum
Meaning: Fifth Born
Gender: Boy

Name: Apace
Meaning: Swift
Gender: Boy

Name: Arabella
Meaning: Beautiful
Gender: Girl

Name: Arden
Meaning: Eagle Valley
Gender: Girl

Name: Arley
Meaning: Of the Meadow
Gender: Boy

Name: Asamoah
Meaning: Unknown
Gender: Boy

Name: Ashon
Meaning: Seventh Son
Gender: Boy

Name: Ata
Meaning: Twin
Gender: Boy

Name: Atiyah
Meaning: Gift
Gender: Girl

Name: Ato
Meaning: Born on Saturday
Gender: Boy

Name: Audree
Meaning: Noble and Strong
Gender: Girl

Name: Azacca
Meaning: Spirit of Agriculture
Gender: Boy

Name: Azhar
Meaning: Luminous
Gender: Girl

Name: Azzam
Meaning: Determined
Gender: Girl

Name: Badrick
Meaning: Ruler
Gender: Boy

Name: Badu
Meaning: Tenth Born
Gender: Girl

Name: Bashirah
Meaning: Bringer of Good Tidings
Gender: Girl

Name: Beaman
Meaning: Beekeeper
Gender: Boy

Name: Bede
Meaning: Prayer
Gender: Boy

Name: Bedu, Baduwaa, Badu
Meaning: Tenth Born
Gender: Boy

Name: Benedicta
Meaning: Blessed
Gender: Girl

Name: Beryl
Meaning: Green Jewel
Gender: Girl

Name: Blakely
Meaning: Dark Meadow
Gender: Boy

Name: Bo
Meaning: Attractive
Gender: Boy

Name: Boahinmaa
Meaning: She will Leave
Gender: Girl

Name: Bodua
Meaning: Animal Tail
Gender: Girl

Name: Botwe
Meaning: Eighth Born
Gender: Boy

Name: Bour
Meaning: Rock
Gender: Girl

Name: Brantley
Meaning: Proud
Gender: Boy

Name: Brawley
Meaning: Hill Dweller
Gender: Boy

Name: Braxton
Meaning: Brock's Town
Gender: Girl

Name: Buckminster
Meaning: Preacher
Gender: Boy

Name: Burdan
Meaning: Valley of Trees
Gender: Boy

Name: Burgess
Meaning: Store Owner
Gender: Boy

Name: Camilla
Meaning: Perfect
Gender: Girl

Name: Cara
Meaning: Dearest
Gender: Girl

Name: Caralyn
Meaning: Small but Strong
Gender: Girl

Name: Caridad
Meaning: Affectionate
Gender: Girl

Name: Carnell
Meaning: Protector of the Castle
Gender: Boy

Name: Carson
Meaning: Son of Carr
Gender: Boy

Name: Cartland
Meaning: Unknown
Gender: Boy

Name: Carver
Meaning: He who Carves Wood
Gender: Boy

Name: Charlaine
Meaning: Strong
Gender: Girl

Name: Chasity
Meaning: Pure
Gender: Girl

Name: Chilton
Meaning: Farm Dweller
Gender: Boy

Name: Chip
Meaning: Farmer
Gender: Boy

Name: Churchill
Meaning: Unknown
Gender: Boy

Name: Clemence
Meaning: Merciful
Gender: Girl

Name: Clover
Meaning: Fortunate
Gender: Girl

Name: Dalbert
Meaning: Bright
Gender: Boy

Name: Dalena
Meaning: Valley
Gender: Girl

Name: Damarae
Meaning: Joy
Gender: Boy

Name: Dana
Meaning: Danish
Gender: Girl

Name: Dante
Meaning: Everlasting
Gender: Boy

Name: Daralis
Meaning: Beloved
Gender: Girl

Name: Delton
Meaning: Valley Town
Gender: Boy

Name: Delwyn
Meaning: Valley Dweller
Gender: Girl

Name: Delyse
Meaning: Delightful
Gender: Girl

Name: Dhakirah
Meaning: Faith in God
Gender: Girl

Name: Do
Meaning: First Born after Twins
Gender: Girl

Name: Dofi
Meaning: Unknown
Gender: Girl

Name: Donkor
Meaning: Humble
Gender: Boy

Name: Duku
Meaning: Eleventh Born
Gender: Boy

Name: Dunu
Meaning: Twelfth Born
Gender: Boy

Name: Drusilla
Meaning: Sturdy
Gender: Girl

Name: Duette
Meaning: Twin
Gender: Girl

Name: Dunton
Meaning: Town on a Hill
Gender: Boy

Name: Durenne
Meaning: Everlasting
Gender: Girl

Name: Durward
Meaning: Gatekeeper
Gender: Boy

Name: Dusty
Meaning: Fighter
Gender: Boy

Name: Dymond
Meaning: Gem
Gender: Girl

Name: Ebo
Meaning: Born on Tuesday
Gender: Boy

Name: Edwina
Meaning: Prosperous
Gender: Girl

Name: Ekow
Meaning: Born on Thursday
Gender: Boy

Name: Eldon
Meaning: Old Farm
Gender: Boy

Name: Eldridge
Meaning: Wise
Gender: Boy

Name: Elgin
Meaning: Noble
Gender: Boy

Name: Ernestina
Meaning: Earnest
Gender: Girl

Name: Esam
Meaning: Safeguard
Gender: Girl

Name: Esi
Meaning: Born on Sunday
Gender: Girl

Name: Essence
Meaning: Life
Gender: Girl

Name: Ethan
Meaning: Strong
Gender: Boy

Name: Evan
Meaning: Little Warrior
Gender: Boy

Name: Evelia
Meaning: Second Born
Gender: Boy

Name: Evelyn
Meaning: Hazelnut
Gender: Boy

Name: Everley
Meaning: Where the Boars Dwell
Gender: Boy

Name: Fadi
Meaning: Redeemer
Gender: Boy

Name: Farhanah
Meaning: Happy
Gender: Girl

Name: Felicity
Meaning: Happy
Gender: Girl

Name: Femi
Meaning: Loved One
Gender: Girl

Name: Fenuku
Meaning: Late Birth
Gender: Girl

Name: Fifi
Meaning: Born on Friday
Gender: Girl

Name: Fiorel
Meaning: Flower
Gender: Girl

Name: Fodjour
Meaning: Fourth Born
Gender: Girl

Name: Fram
Meaning: Ofram Tree
Gender: Girl

Name: Fuller
Meaning: Thick
Gender: Boy

Name: Garnet
Meaning: Red Gem
Gender: Girl

Name: Gayla
Meaning: Lively
Gender: Girl

Name: Gayna
Meaning: Phantom
Gender: Girl

Name: Gerome
Meaning: Holy
Gender: Boy

Name: Gerrod
Meaning: Spearman
Gender: Boy

Name: Gharam
Meaning: Love
Gender: Girl

Name: Ghassan
Meaning: Unknown
Gender: Boy

Name: Ghazi
Meaning: Conqueror
Gender: Girl

Name: Gifford
Meaning: Generous
Gender: Boy

Name: Goldie
Meaning: Golden
Gender: Girl

Name: Gracie
Meaning: Graceful
Gender: Girl

Name: Grover
Meaning: From the Groves
Gender: Boy

Name: Gyasi
Meaning: Wonderful
Gender: Girl

Name: Hadley
Meaning: Meadow
Gender: Boy

Name: Hani-Ah
Meaning: Bliss
Gender: Girl

Name: Haytham
Meaning: Young Hawk
Gender: Boy

Name: Heaven
Meaning: Eternally Happy
Gender: Girl

Name: Henna
Meaning: Ruler of the Home
Gender: Girl

Name: Hilal
Meaning: Happiness
Gender: Girl

Name: Hollis
Meaning: Holly Tree Grove
Gender: Boy

Name: Huda
Meaning: Guide
Gender: Girl

Name: Ife
Meaning: Love
Gender: Boy

Name: Ikhlas
Meaning: Sincere
Gender: Girl

Name: Imo
Meaning: Knowledge
Gender: Boy

Name: Iria
Meaning: Lady
Gender: Girl

Name: Ivy
Meaning: Ivy Tree
Gender: Girl

Name: Jabbar
Meaning: Mighty
Gender: Boy

Name: Jabir
Meaning: Consoler
Gender: Girl

Name: Jaherna
Meaning: Watched by the Lord
Gender: Boy

Name: Jas
Meaning: Supplanter
Gender: Boy

Name: Javaris
Meaning: Spearman
Gender: Boy

Name: Jaxon
Meaning: Son of Jack
Gender: Boy

Name: Jeff
Meaning: Peaceful
Gender: Boy

Name: Jill
Meaning: Youthful
Gender: Girl

Name: Jo
Meaning: God will Provide
Gender: Girl

Name: Joann
Meaning: God is Gracious
Gender: Girl

Name: Jojo
Meaning: Born on Monday
Gender: Girl

Name: Juhanah
Meaning: Young Girl
Gender: Girl

Name: Kady
Meaning: Pure
Gender: Girl

Name: Kakra
Meaning: Younger Twin
Gender: Girl

Name: Kareem
Meaning: Distinguished
Gender: Boy

Name: Kaseem
Meaning: Divided
Gender: Boy

Name: Kayin
Meaning: Long Awaited Child
Gender: Boy

Name: Kayode
Meaning: Bringer of Joy
Gender: Boy

Name: Keldon
Meaning: Port Town
Gender: Boy

Name: Kendra
Meaning: Powerful
Gender: Girl

Name: Kenise
Meaning: Lovely
Gender: Girl

Name: Kesse
Meaning: Large Baby
Gender: Girl

Name: Khenan
Meaning: Rising Sun
Gender: Boy

Name: Kifah
Meaning: Born during Struggle
Gender: Girl

Name: Kim
Meaning: Hollow
Gender: Boy

Name: Kinsey
Meaning: Royal Kin
Gender: Boy

Name: Kisi
Meaning: Born on Sunday
Gender: Girl

Name: Kobby, Kobina
Meaning: Born on Tuesday
Gender: Boy

Name: Kontar
Meaning: Only Child
Gender: Girl

Name: Kpodo
Meaning: Elder Twin
Gender: Boy

Name: Kukua
Meaning: Born on Wednesday
Gender: Girl

Name: Kunto
Meaning: Third Born
Gender: Girl

Name: Kyere
Meaning: Unknown
Gender: Girl

Name: Kyler
Meaning: Unknown
Gender: Boy

Name: Kyndal
Meaning: Valley Ruler
Gender: Girl

Name: Kyndra
Meaning: Born of the Water
Gender: Girl

Name: Landon
Meaning: Meadow
Gender: Girl

Name: Laurie
Meaning: Crowned with Laurel
Gender: Boy

Name: Leigh
Meaning: Poetic
Gender: Girl

Name: Leoma
Meaning: Intelligent
Gender: Girl

Name: Libano
Meaning: Fair Skinned
Gender: Boy

Name: Liber
Meaning: Bringer of Abundance
Gender: Boy

Name: Lizabeth
Meaning: Consecrated to God
Gender: Girl

Name: London
Meaning: Moon Fortress
Gender: Girl

Name: Lora
Meaning: Crowned with Laurel
Gender: Girl

Name: Lorimer
Meaning: Unknown
Gender: Boy

Name: Loritz
Meaning: Laurel
Gender: Boy

Name: Lu'lu
Meaning: Pearls
Gender: Girl

Name: Lumo
Meaning: Long Delivery
Gender: Boy

Name: Lumusi
Meaning: Unknown
Gender: Girl

Name: Lyndon
Meaning: Linden Tree Hill
Gender: Boy

Name: Lynnell
Meaning: Beautiful
Gender: Girl

Name: Lyron
Meaning: Song
Gender: Boy

Name: Mabel
Meaning: Loveable
Gender: Girl

Name: Majid
Meaning: Glorious
Gender: Girl

Name: Malik
Meaning: Sovereign
Gender: Boy

Name: Malikah
Meaning: Queen
Gender: Girl

Name: Mama
Meaning: Born on Saturday
Gender: Girl

Name: Manu, Maanu
Meaning: Second Born
Gender: Boy

Name: Maresa
Meaning: Of the Sea
Gender: Girl

Name: Marge
Meaning: Pearl
Gender: Girl

Name: Martisha
Meaning: Martial
Gender: Girl

Name: Marty
Meaning: Sorrowful
Gender: Girl

Name: Marvelle
Meaning: Awe and Wonder
Gender: Girl

Name: Masel
Meaning: Unknown
Gender: Boy

Name: Matt
Meaning: Gift from God
Gender: Boy

Name: Maven
Meaning: Wise
Gender: Boy

Name: Mawulawde
Meaning: God will Provide
Gender: Boy

Name: Mawuli
Meaning: There is a God
Gender: Boy

Name: Mawusi
Meaning: In the Hands of God
Gender: Girl

Name: Mayyasah
Meaning: Walks with Pride
Gender: Girl

Name: Miles
Meaning: Merciful
Gender: Boy

Name: Millard
Meaning: Miller
Gender: Boy

Name: Millicent
Meaning: Industrious
Gender: Girl

Name: Morowa
Meaning: Royal
Gender: Girl

Name: Msrah
Meaning: Sixth Born
Gender: Boy

Name: Mushirah
Meaning: Advisor
Gender: Girl

Name: Naim
Meaning: Tranquility
Gender: Boy

Name: Najla
Meaning: Wide Eyed
Gender: Girl

Name: Nana
Meaning: Mother of Earth
Gender: Girl

Name: Nanyamka
Meaning: Gift from God
Gender: Girl

Name: Newman
Meaning: Newcomer
Gender: Boy

Name: Nibras
Meaning: Light
Gender: Girl

Name: Nida
Meaning: Our Call
Gender: Girl

Name: Nollie
Meaning: Blossoming Flower
Gender: Girl

Name: Nsoah
Meaning: Seventh Born
Gender: Boy

Name: Num
Meaning: Fifth Born
Gender: Boy

Name: Nyamekye
Meaning: God's Gift
Gender: Boy

Name: Odom
Meaning: Oak Tree
Gender: Boy

Name: Ogden
Meaning: Oak Valley
Gender: Boy

Name: Ojise
Meaning: Angel
Gender: Boy

Name: Oko
Meaning: Eldest Twin
Gender: Boy

Name: Olukayode
Meaning: God Brings Happiness
Gender: Boy

Name: Olumide
Meaning: God has Come
Gender: Boy

Name: Omnira
Meaning: Liberated
Gender: Girl

Name: Ora
Meaning: Prayer
Gender: Girl

Name: Osei
Meaning: Noble
Gender: Boy

Name: Owusu
Meaning: Unknown
Gender: Boy

Name: Ozigbodi
Meaning: Long Awaited For
Gender: Girl

Name: Panyin
Meaning: Eldest Twin
Gender: Girl

Name: Perry
Meaning: Falcon
Gender: Boy

Name: Pipina
Meaning: God will Provide
Gender: Girl

Name: Pippa
Meaning: Lover of Horses
Gender: Girl

Name: Placencia
Meaning: Pleasant
Gender: Girl

Name: Prah
Meaning: River
Gender: Boy

Name: Qadriyah
Meaning: God's Will
Gender: Girl

Name: Qamar
Meaning: Born during a Full Moon
Gender: Girl

Name: Qasim
Meaning: Distributor
Gender: Boy

Name: Ra'idah
Meaning: Leader
Gender: Girl

Name: Ra'ifah
Meaning: Merciful
Gender: Girl

Name: Rad
Meaning: Advisor
Gender: Boy

Name: Raeni
Meaning: Queen
Gender: Girl

Name: Randee
Meaning: Protected
Gender: Girl

Name: Raveen
Meaning: Blackbird
Gender: Girl

Name: Rayce
Meaning: Swift
Gender: Boy

Name: Raymon
Meaning: Protector
Gender: Boy

Name: Read
Meaning: Red Hair
Gender: Boy

Name: Riham
Meaning: Everlasting
Gender: Girl

Name: Rihana
Meaning: Basil
Gender: Girl

Name: Rockland
Meaning: Land of Rocks
Gender: Boy

Name: Romola
Meaning: From Italy
Gender: Girl

Name: Ronica
Meaning: Honest
Gender: Girl

Name: Ros, Rosalie
Meaning: Rose
Gender: Girl

Name: Ryder
Meaning: Horsemen
Gender: Boy

Name: Sabir
Meaning: Patient
Gender: Boy

Name: Sa'dah
Meaning: Happiness
Gender: Girl

Name: Sa'diyah
Meaning: Fortunate
Gender: Girl

Name: Sabreena
Meaning: Princess
Gender: Girl

Name: Sage
Meaning: Wise
Gender: Girl

Name: Samihah
Meaning: Generous
Gender: Girl

Name: Samirah
Meaning: Companion
Gender: Girl

Name: Sebastian
Meaning: Revered
Gender: Boy

Name: Serwa
Meaning: Noble
Gender: Girl

Name: Shafiq
Meaning: Compassionate
Gender: Boy

Name: Shams
Meaning: Sun
Gender: Girl

Name: Shandi
Meaning: God is Gracious
Gender: Girl

Name: Sharee
Meaning: Dear One
Gender: Girl

Name: Sharifah
Meaning: Noble
Gender: Girl

Name: Siisi
Meaning: Born on Sunday
Gender: Boy

Name: Sono
Meaning: Elephant
Gender: Boy

Name: Stacia
Meaning: Resurrection
Gender: Girl

Name: Stanwick
Meaning: Stony Village
Gender: Boy

Name: Starleen
Meaning: Star
Gender: Girl

Name: Starling
Meaning: Singing Bird
Gender: Girl

Name: Stowe
Meaning: Unknown
Gender: Boy

Name: Stroud
Meaning: Thicket
Gender: Boy

Name: Tacey
Meaning: Gazelle
Gender: Girl

Name: Taite
Meaning: Cheery
Gender: Girl

Name: Tandie
Meaning: Team
Gender: Boy

Name: Taniyah
Meaning: Joyous
Gender: Girl

Name: Tano
Meaning: From the Water
Gender: Boy

Name: Tasnim
Meaning: Born in Paradise
Gender: Girl

Name: Tawbah
Meaning: Unknown
Gender: Girl

Name: Tayla
Meaning: Tailor
Gender: Girl

Name: Thel
Meaning: Unknown
Gender: Boy

Name: Thema
Meaning: Queen
Gender: Girl

Name: Toller
Meaning: Collector
Gender: Boy

Name: Torey
Meaning: Tower
Gender: Boy

Name: Tse
Meaning: Youngest Twin
Gender: Boy

Name: Twia
Meaning: Brother of Twins
Gender: Boy

Name: Tyne
Meaning: River
Gender: Girl

Name: Ubadah
Meaning: Servant of God
Gender: Boy

Name: Vance
Meaning: From the Marsh
Gender: Boy

Name: Vea
Meaning: Seen
Gender: Girl

Name: Veruca
Meaning: Unknown
Gender: Girl

Name: Viktoria
Meaning: Victorious
Gender: Girl

Name: Virtudes
Meaning: Blessed Spirit
Gender: Girl

Name: Vivian
Meaning: Lively
Gender: Girl

Name: Wafaa
Meaning: Faithful
Gender: Girl

Name: Wafiqah
Meaning: Successful
Gender: Girl

Name: Ware
Meaning: Cautious
Gender: Boy

Name: Willie
Meaning: Guardian
Gender: Girl

Name: Willow
Meaning: Tree
Gender: Girl

Name: Wylie
Meaning: Charming
Gender: Boy

Name: Wyman
Meaning: Warrior
Gender: Boy

Name: Yaa, Yaaba, Yaaya
Meaning: Born on Thursday
Gender: Girl

Name: Yafeu
Meaning: Bold
Gender: Boy

Name: Yakootah
Meaning: Emerald
Gender: Girl

Name: Yamha
Meaning: Dove
Gender: Girl

Name: Yao
Meaning: Born on Thursday
Gender: Boy

Name: Yasin
Meaning: Muhammad
Gender: Boy

Name: Ye
Meaning: Eldest Twin
Gender: Girl

Name: Zuhrah
Meaning: Bright
Gender: Girl